Fix Your Dig Fast

THE AYURVEDIC METHOD WITH VERY FEW BIG WORDS AND NO FLUFF

Based on the knowledge of Āyurveda

Copyright of Gopi Ayurveda ltd. © 2025. All rights reserved.

No part of this publication may be copied, reproduced in any format, by any means, electronic or otherwise, without prior consent from the copyright owner and publisher of this book.

By Maxim Bishop

Contents

Introduction 3

Digestive Fire 9

Only eat when you're hungry 12

Chew your food. More 19

Don't eat too much 25

Eat at the same time everyday 31

Burps are your secret weapon 34

Don't eat at night 37

Good sleep 40

Food as a medicine 42

Battle with your mind 44

1. Introduction.

"Nothing wrecks your day faster than bad digestion"

– Me.

Nothing wrecks your day faster than bad digestion.
You feel tired, bloated, and irritable. Your skin flares up. Your head fogs over.
It kills your focus, your mood, your drive — everything.

I wrote this book because that was me.
In 2020, my skin was so raw I couldn't sleep. I tried every cream, cleanse, and miracle hack I could find. Nothing lasted.
Then I stumbled into Ayurveda.

What is Āyurveda?

Āyurveda is common sense.
Eat when you're hungry. Chew your food. Rest when you're tired. Simple. Intuitive. But it works, and fast.

It's the oldest knowledge of health and medicine in the world. It's scriptures date back up to 5000 years, coded in the ancient Sanskrit language. It's passed down through millennia. It's passed down through great sages in the Himalayan mountains, to your Grandma's kitchen.

Really. You'll notice a lot of what I say is what you may have shrugged off as "things your grandma used to say."

Āyurveda aims at the *roots* of our health problems rather than only treating the symptoms. Āyurveda is the science of understanding how our bodies work in harmony with nature.

There's a whole lot more to Āyurveda than what I cover here. It's a rich body of knowledge. And I will be making more books to explain other important topics in the same easy-to-understand way.

This book helps people understand the fundamentals of Āyurveda and make changes in their lives in a day.

Of course, you'll have to do the work.

This book isn't a medical manual. It's a practical guide to principles that have helped countless generations of people feel lighter, clearer, and more alive. It's a short book. But that's only because I *hate* fluff. I don't want to waste your time and mine.

It won't fix everything overnight, but it's a start.
And the payout? *Massive*.

First, a little story.

I was talking to a stranger on London Bridge in the middle of the day sometime in the middle of the summer of 2020. During our discussion, he noticed a little red patch of dry skin on my neck.

"What's that?" He pointed to my neck with a facial expression that was a mixture of disgust and concern.

"What's what?" I had absolutely no idea what he was talking about.

"You got some eczema or something on your neck."

I felt around my neck, looking for what he was pointing to. Then I felt it. Dry. Small. And when I touched it, it became itchy and stung a little.

I headed home. I didn't think much of it at the time.

But 2 weeks later…

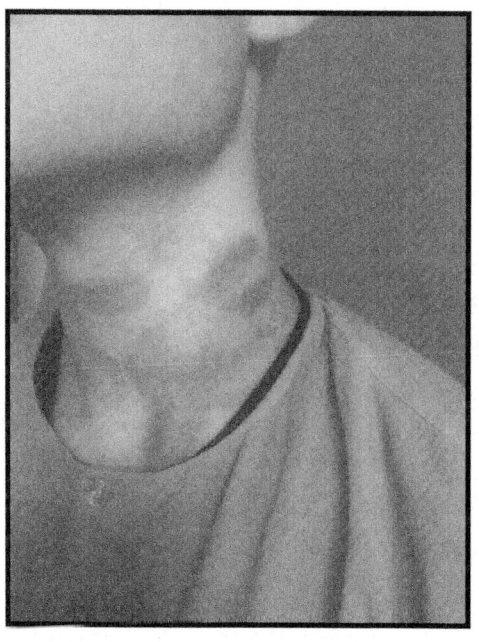

There she is…

Well, that escalated quickly.

The next six months were *hell*. I spent countless nights waking up in the middle of sleep. I found my fingers scratching my neck, covered in blood and pus.

If you decided to eat something while reading this, I am *so* sorry.

Creams, detoxes, *honey*. You name it; if it was meant to help eczema, I tried it.

And none of it did anything.

Frustrated, and very itchy, I decided to investigate the root cause of eczema. I had followed what various websites told me to do for long enough.

I noticed that everyone was recommending topical products. That means they go on top of the skin.

Everything was just treating the symptoms.

It wasn't too long before I learned that there is some theory that eczema starts from the gut. A history of poor gut health means a buildup of toxins that eventually starts to leak out of the skin. (By the way, this isn't medical advice, and I'm not claiming to be a medical professional or expert. But, all I'm saying is nothing made sense or worked for me until I found this out).

"Oh, I gotta work on the *inside*," I thought to myself. I had spent so much time, money, and energy focusing on the outside. It had never crossed my mind that there might be more than meets the eye.

I started doing some cleanses with lemon juice. I made a

purgation drink using orange juice and castor oil. Purgation is a strong laxative that clears the bowels.. I tried fasting for 2 weeks without any food.

Yes.

By March of 2021, the eczema had already made its way down to my chest. Red patches covered half of my torso.

I was ready to try anything.

And it started to work.

By April of 2021, the eczema had pretty much cleared. I could sleep in peace. The bleeding and pus stopped.

To finish it off, I rubbed mustard oil on top of the stubborn infected patches that remained. It stung like *hellfire*. But the next day, would you believe it, it had cleared up.

6 months of terrible, embarrassing pain. Now it was over. I was free. And I had learned some lessons that changed the course of my life.

Discovering the importance of digestive health inspired me to research Āyurveda. Āyurveda stresses the importance of internal health and good habits rather than medication. After fixing my eczema by focusing on digestion, I realised Āyurveda was onto something.

And now, I'll share that something.

Who is this book for?

The problem with most digestive health advice out there is that it is

a) made up

b) requires you to buy something like a pill, juice, fruit or vegetable, powder, etc.,

or c) only tells you *what* to eat rather than *how* to eat.

Some advice is borderline *lethal*. (Like drinking 8 glasses of water per day regardless of whether you're thirsty)

If you're lucky enough to find something about Āyurveda, it can seem broad, confusing, and packed with tricky Sanskrit terms.

Āyurveda is huge. And very helpful in all aspects of health. But sometimes you just want to know all the ways you can fix your digestion. For free. Without buying any fancy herbs. Or changing *what* you eat.

That's who this book is for.

Also, it will help you save money, which is a nice bonus.

1. Digestive Fire.

"Good digestion waits on appetite, and health on both"

- William Shakspeare

> ## Digestive Fire Math
>
> 🗨 = 🔥
>
> your Stomach is a fire
>
> 🔥 + ❄ = ⃠
>
> Fire and cold don't mix
>
> 🔥 + 💧 = ⃠
>
> fire and too much water don't mix
>
> 🔥 + 🪵 = ⃠
>
> fire and too much wood don't mix

The Āyurvedic scriptures call it *agni* (literally, fire). In modern terms we call it acid. Āyurveda compares digestion with fire to make things easy. t likes this name better than "acid" since "acid" doesn't show us how to keep our digestion healthy.

Here's why.

When you're hungry, it does feel like you have a fire in your stomach. Your digestion works alot like a fire because it burns up food. Food can be compared to wood. Wood is a fuel for fire, and we use that fire to see and to be warm. In other words, fire helps us survive.

So, we should keep our fire lit to survive and *thrive*. Because you *can* live without fire, at least for some time. But it will be difficult and unpleasant.

In the same way, you can live without keeping your digestion healthy. But you will live for a lot less time. And throughout your life, you'll experience more disease. According to Āyurveda.

How to keep the fire going

Balancing the fire within our bellies is easy. It works like any other fire.

Fire should be burning before adding more wood. If you add wood before the fire is burning, it will never start.

If you eat before you're hungry, your small digestive fire won't handle the load of food. Then, the food sits in your stomach. The Sushruta Samhita (an Āyurvedic text) says that this is one of the causes of obesity.

If you put too much wood on a fire, the fire will go out then, too. The same applies inside the body. Overeating (More detail on this later in the book) is like putting too much wood on a fire. The flames just get suffocated, and you can't use the fire for heat and light anymore. Ever wonder why you feel so tired after a stuffing meal? You extinguished your fire.

The stomach acid is like fire and works in a way like fire. So, things that generate heat, in moderation, aid digestion. In practice, this means exercise is useful for boosting digestive strength. But only up to the point of sweat on the forehead, as any more produces too much heat. A machine gets hot with repeated movement, and our body's a machine. Movement makes heat. That heat fuels digestion.

If a fire is too strong, though, you could burn yourself. The Āyurveda recommends avoiding too much spicy food for this reason. We often call spicy food "hot". That's because it heats up our mouths and the rest of our bodies. Spicy food increases the fire in your stomach, which is good in moderation for burning wood. But in excess, the fire can get out of control and burn you. Ever wonder why heartburn and acid reflux feel so fiery? They happen because of too much digestive fire, a result of too many chilies or other heating spices.

Some morning sun (afternoon sun is not recommended) also boosts digestion. The sun *is* a big ball of fire, after all.

Naturally, cold food will slow your fire. Ice creams and iced drinks, except on very hot days, are not recommended.

There are many more details about your digestive fire that we won't cover in this book. Āyurveda is a big science. The rest of the book will show you how Āyurveda can boost your wellbeing and digestion, without the complicated details.

2. Only eat when you're hungry.

"I saw few die of hunger; of eating, a hundred thousand."

- Benjamin Franklin

If you can master this, everything else is easy.

It sounds kind of stupid, right? We know that hunger means we should eat.

But at the same time, many of us eat when we are not hungry. We eat because some diet fad tells us to eat at a certain time, not because our body does. Or we feel like snacking. We're at a family event and there's food served, so we're obliged. In other words, there are many times we eat before we need to.

Eating before you're hungry can make your body feel heavy or uncomfortable later. This is because your body isn't ready to digest the food.

Plus, you don't get half or barely any of the nutrients you need. Toxins build up because the undigested food stores itself in the body.

That's a major reason why we get diseased, according to Āyurveda.

Āyurveda calls those built-up toxins āmā. This toxic waste pollutes our whole body and slows down our organs.

A note on āma

The toxic goo that fills up your body is much like soot in a chimney, gunk in a pipe, or build-up in a drain. The difference between āmā and these examples is that if you keep your digestion strong, it never has to build up. The fire of digestion will keep the bodies pathways clear. According to Āyurveda, the body has pathways for nutrients, blood, air, and even thoughts. When these get blocked, you feel it. So, āmā is a critical aspect to this whole digestion thing. Think of āmā as the bad guy in your heroic fight to get back your health.

Digestion is the process of breaking food down into nutrients. If we don't manage the fire well, our body doesn't get the nutrients that we bought the food for in the first place.

And yes, that does mean you should skip a meal if you don't feel hungry at your usual time for eating. Because it's better to skip than to eat on a stomach that isn't ready.

People often put so much emphasis on *what* to eat. But very few talk about *how* to eat. Without a strong fire, nothing burns.

The financial loss of eating before we're hungry.

You are *throwing* money away.

Food usually costs money. And we earn money partly to buy food. We buy food knowing that it keeps us alive. That's the whole point of food, right? But when digestion is poor, we struggle to absorb food. It just turns into āmā (toxins). This can lead to weakness in our body from toxins and not enough nutrition. As a result, there is disease. So, most of the money spent on food is *creating* disease. Unless we fix our digestion.

The average monthly cost of groceries in the United Kingdom is £715 per household. We can guess that only 20% of your food is digested when you don't follow Āyurvedic wisdom. That means the average household wastes £6,864 a year on undigested food.

Snacking

Snacking before your last meal digests means your body has to switch focus. Instead of digesting the previous meal, it starts on the new food you just ate. The last meal sits in your stomach, causing bloating, heaviness, and toxic buildup. And even if you just eat a little bit, it doesn't get digested well.

So, when should we eat?

Wait until your mind can't stop thinking about food. That's your body saying: "your fire's ready."

If we are even prepared to enact *physical violence* to get food, that's the right time to eat. This doesn't mean you should starve yourself. But if you think you're hungry, wait thirty minutes. See if that rumbling in your tummy keeps burning. Because it may just be some bowel movements mistaken as hunger.

When you time your meals right, you learn when you're usually hungry and when you pass waste.

In general, hunger comes *after* bowel movements. The

intestine is part of the digestive process; it absorbs nutrients. The whole process of passing waste is the final phase of digestion. So, only when you poo is your body ready for another meal. Then, your body will let you know. "Now you can eat. I'm ready." Think about a normal fire. Fire requires oxygen for it to burn. It needs air. So, there should be space in your digestive system for air to flow freely. Then the fire can burn. When the poo leaves your bowels, there is more space for air to flow.

When in doubt…

If you have a doubt, the best is to avoid eating. If you ask, "Am I really hungry?" it's not the time yet.

So, I have a short story about this.

My wife wanted to eat something only a couple hours after her previous meal, so I knew that she couldn't possibly be hungry. It was much more likely to be a craving, which is very different.

So, I just asked her, "are you sure you're hungry?"

She didn't quickly answer yes or no. She looked up and thought for a few moments.

Before she even had time to say "yes," I stopped her and said, "that means you are not ready. The very fact you thought about it means you can wait some more."

She smiled.

Following this is the first crucial step to digestive health. It's the most important thing. Without hunger, no other rule matters.

Wait till you're thirsty

Water is trickier.

Because water and fire are opposites, Āyurveda advises drinking water carefully. In Āyurveda, a long list of problems in your health is because:

a) you drink water when you're not thirsty

b) you take too much,

c) you chug it (instead of sipping) during eating and in general, and

d) It's too darn cold.

Cold water (God forbid *ice* water) is opposite to fire, which has the quality of heat.

Cold and heat are opposites. See how it's easy to understand?

Āyurveda.

Like hunger, thirst is the body's way of telling us it's time to drink. We get thirsty when there is a healthy digestive fire. Fire tends to evaporate water.

Pretty simple stuff. Listen to your body.

What about the taste?

Why do we eat in the first place, after all? Or drink water?

It's to keep us alive.

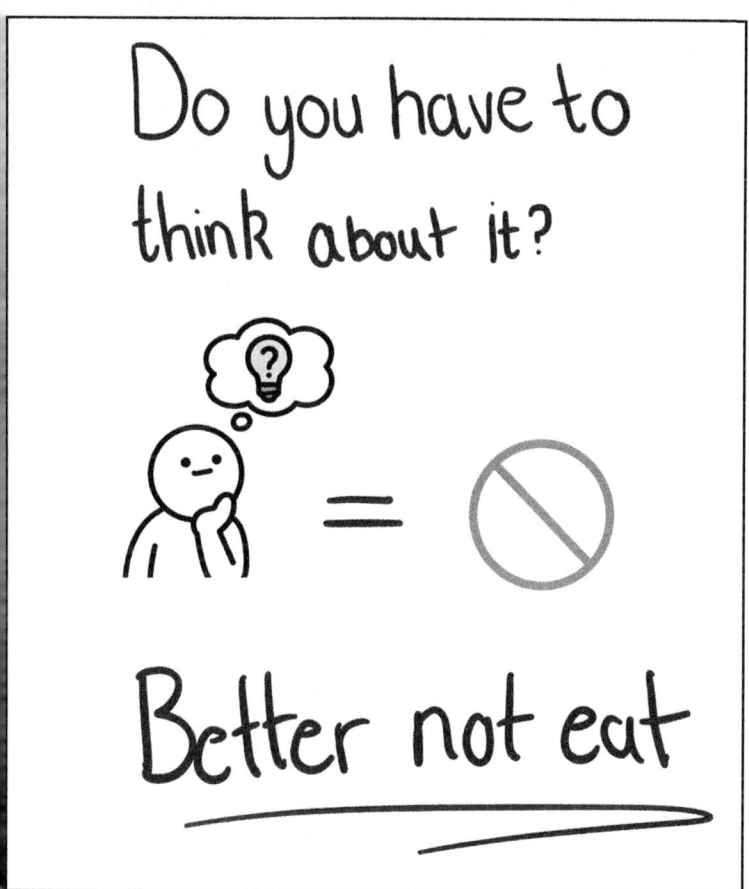

So, if we are not ready to digest, why should we eat? If we're not thirsty, it's not time to drink.

You were probably taught to drink oh-so-many litres of water every day. Then again, do you still believe in Santa Claus? Not everything we learned as a child is true.

You might argue that eating is for taste. And after all, taste is another demand of the body. Like our stomach is asking for food, our tongue is asking for taste.

No disagreement there. Taste is a wonderful thing. It's something that motivates us to eat. But it isn't the *main* thing.

If you don't eat, you *die*. But even if food doesn't *taste* great, you can still live. So, the difference between eating and taste is the difference between *life and death*.

Taste is nice but not needed. It's like salt. You can eat anything without salt. But salt makes food taste better. But if it's poison on your plate, no matter how tasty it is with some salt, you shouldn't eat it.

Eating food before you're hungry is akin to eating poison, says Āyurveda.

That's it — the first rule. Eat when hungry; drink when thirsty.

Sounds obvious, but most of modern life trains us to ignore those signals. That's a curious thing, isn't it? Why should we ignore the natural signs our body sends us?

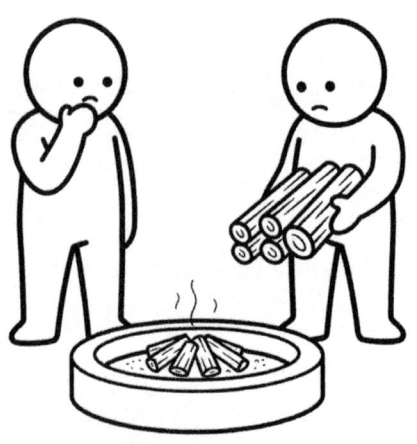

"I don't think that's gonna work..."

3. Chew your food. More.

"Don't eat fast food. Eat food slowly." - Me. Again.

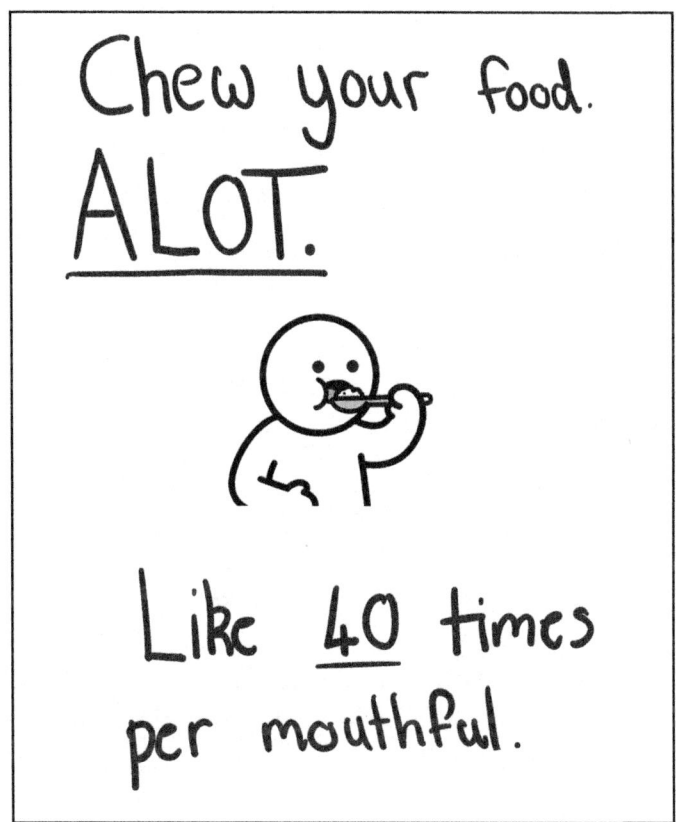

Everyone knows we must chew our food. But they generally don't know *how much* to chew. Spoiler: *it's a lot.*

Like, each mouthful around 40 times.

It's *that* much.

To make this obvious, think for a sec about why we chew. It's so we can swallow and digest the food. Trying to swallow a whole apple without chewing would be dangerous. It might be your last meal unless someone knows the Heimlich manoeuvre. In other words, you'll choke.

Chewing makes it easier for our bodies to accept food. By extension of that logic, the more we chew, the easier the food is to digest.

You can practise this, and it will take some concentration. Most of us, as I say, generally *breathe* in our food. We *inhale* it. Much like a vacuum cleaner. Especially if we're in a rush.

So, usually, we don't chew our food very much. But that leads to lots of large bits of food. The stomach doesn't handle those as well as your teeth do.

The power of teeth

Your teeth are a lot more powerful than your stomach. You have teeth for a reason. Please use them. They're not only for showing how beautiful you are. When you eat a meal, it will take at least 4 hours (depending on what and how you eat) to digest.

But if you chew something, it's broken down to a liquid in less than a minute. The teeth can do a lot of hard work for you. Think about the difference in time there. Sure, the food is ideally broken down already when it reaches your stomach. But four hours? That's a *huge* difference.

Chewing more gives you a better return on investment than letting your stomach do the work. It will take longer to digest down there, and you'll lose more energy.

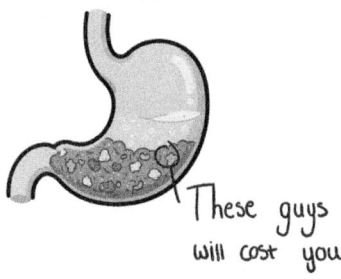

Because digestion burns energy. Energy, mostly in the form of blood flow, is required by your stomach. If the food is difficult to break down because you don't chew enough, you lose more energy. If you make the job easy for the stomach, your body spends less energy on digestion.

Ayurveda teaches that digestion begins in the mouth Food is meant to change from solid to liquid. According to the Āyurveda, the body has an easier time processing liquid food. A towel absorbs water significantly better than it does a potato. Because the pores and fibers of the towel are very fine, solid food cannot enter them.

That was a weird analogy.

But you get the point; your cells that absorb the food are also very fine, so they absorb a liquid state of food better. It takes quite some time to chew food to a liquid. It takes *conscious* effort to move from chewing your food enough for you to swallow to making it a liquid.

In fact, it can be borderline *annoying* to chew your food

so much. But when you see the difference in how light you feel afterwards, you'll never second-guess it again. You can test this by trying to swallow food you hardly chew. Your gag reflex will likely reject it. You'll cough, choke, etc.

Chewing is important. Chew more. Chew till there's nothing solid in your mouth.

A numbers game

If you crunch the numbers, it seems in the beginning to be not worth the time to chew more. Let's say your average amount of chews is 10. It might take you 15 seconds. If you increase your chews to the recommended 40, it takes roughly 2.5 times longer.

And so, if your average mealtime is 10 minutes, it'll now take you 25.

That seems like a lot of time lost.

Āyurveda poses an interesting question: if you can trade an extra hour each day for decades more of life, is that not a valuable investment? With much less disease later, it seems worth it.

Bonuses compound too. Your quality of life improves not just later, but also while you practice chewing more. You absorb more nutrients, which helps you become stronger and healthier.

Also, you experience less pain related to digestion.

Plus, Āyurveda suggests that we feel sleepier when toxins are in our bodies and digestion isn't good. So, 15 minutes extra per meal could possibly save you hours in the bed.

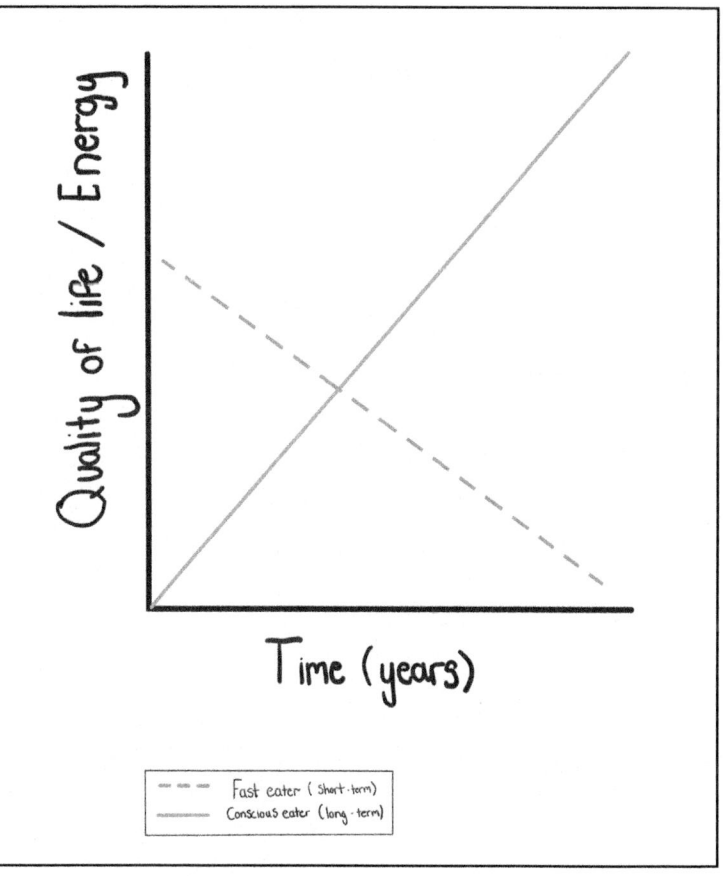

The dotted graph starts higher because if you don't focus on chewing so much, eating is easier. As you can see though, it's not worth the trade.

Worth a thought.

In other words, you're not only investing in your future, but your present life quality standard goes up.

Seems like a good deal now, right?

Chew more → Absorb more

Better absorption → More energy

More energy → Stronger digestion

Fewer illnesses → Longer, happier life

4. Don't eat too much.

"Everything in excess is opposed to nature" – Hippocrates

Food is amazing. I get it. I agree with you. But if you eat too much, your stomach struggles to digest. And when your body crashes, half the menu is off-limits. It's best to enjoy in smaller amounts rather than to avoid it for long or to overeat at once.

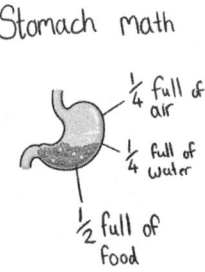

Āyurveda is simple: fill half your stomach with food, a quarter with water, and leave a quarter empty for air and movement. Water is to help move the nutrients throughout the body, and so is air.

Now, you might be thinking, "How on earth do I measure the capacity of my stomach, since it is inside my body?"

Good question. You are very intelligent.

Hold both of your hands out together. Curl the fingers a little bit, cupping them, and keeping them close together. The amount of food you can keep in the little 'hand bowl' you made for yourself now is how much you can take. It's roughly the size of your stomach.

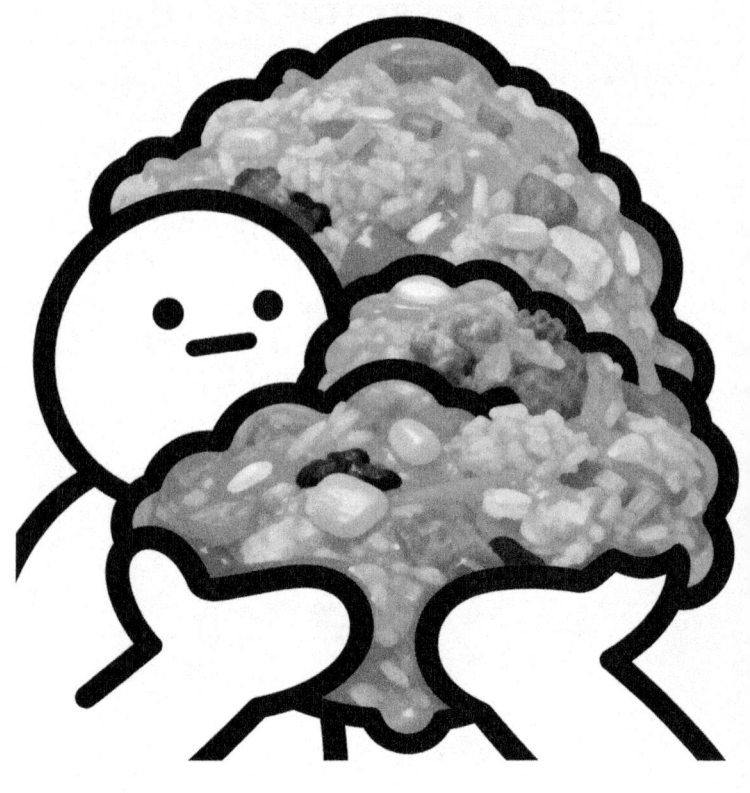

That's... not what I meant

A simple way to stick to this ratio is to eat *half* of what you think you can. Then, drink a bit of water to fill the rest.

The best part of this technique is that you feel its effects right away. You'll notice it the first time you try, and each time after that. Before, you may have felt bloated and sluggish. It was like a small being inside your lower abdomen was stretching your intestines. I couldn't think of a better way to put it. Sorry.

But if you try these ratio tricks, that little fella will be gone the same day. You'll notice a lighter, easier feeling almost immediately. Neato.

Not an easy job.

This is one of, if not *the* hardest rules to follow.

Imagine you have a plate full of delicious food. Imagine you spent *money* on it. Or your mother cooked your old favourite dish for you.

Imagine you're halfway through, and suddenly you burp violently. This matters, and we'll discuss why in chapter 6. At that point, you might feel you shouldn't eat more. You feel the tension in your stomach; the kind that signals pre-indigestion.

Looking down at your plate of delicious food, and then up again at your grandma's sweet face, she asks, "Finish it, dear."

Pure evil, Grandma.

Now you feel obliged to finish that plate.

But you *should not*.

No matter how nice grandma made it. Or how much money you spent.

You can always take it later. But the effect of overeating now will be inescapable, and you *will* feel it later. Not with some discomfort or even pain from indigestion. Not just with tiredness throughout the rest of the day. Not even with grogginess the next morning.

It will strike later as a horrible disease. According to

Āyurveda.

Let's say you're making yourself some toast in the morning. Now, you might think to yourself, "Wow, I'm so hungry; I could go for 2 slices!"

But (sorry to be a party pooper), you should take one slice.

After all, you can always eat the other slice afterwards if you're still hungry. The thing is, the old saying about our eyes being bigger than our stomachs is true for many of us. That in mind, we shouldn't trust what we *think* we can eat. Your mind is not the one who has to digest it, after all. For all that rascal cares, he could take five more servings...

The five stages of digestion.

To keep overeating at bay while in the act of eating, focus on how your stomach feels. Here's how the stomach communicates:

1. Hungry.

2. Getting satisfied.

3. Just right — no hunger, no heaviness.

4. Full.

5. Regret. Bloating. Pain.

At the beginning of the meal, you'll likely feel hungry (if you followed my previous advice). Now, that feeling will go away as you eat. When it reaches the point when you feel neither hungry nor full, it's best to stop eating here.

The slightest sign of fullness, tension in the stomach, is a sign that you are pushing it. Mild discomfort or pain are degrees of indigestion.

Āyurveda suggests eating mindfully. This means avoiding distractions, rushing, or walking while you eat. It's important to pay attention to how you feel while eating. (bonus tip; walking while eating is a very bad idea. The blood is flowing through your legs and can't go to the stomach easily. So, your stomach is slow can't digest well.)

When the air in our stomach is balanced, it flows freely to other parts of the body. This gives us energy and helps us focus. Good airflow also controls the movement of our arms, legs, organs, and thoughts. According to Āyurveda, when air in the stomach is disturbed, other functions in the body can also feel out of balance.

It *is* tough to follow this rule, especially when we like the taste of something. This is where discipline kicks in. Don't worry—it will soon be automatic, like breathing.

You have to think to yourself, "Do I *need* to eat this? Is it worth it for how I will feel after?"

In most cases, the answer is a *resounding* no. After all, you can always take more when you get hungry again.

What if I feel I'm not gaining anything by changing my eating habits?

Look, you don't lose anything here. Because I'm not telling you to *stop eating*. There's not much difference between 2 pancakes and 3 pancakes. You're still going to taste the pancake. And you won't be hungry.

Hopefully you won't be angry about this

Helping others for nothing in return is one of the most fulfilling things you can do. That in mind, I have one question for you.

I can only help people with their digestion using Ayurveda if I can reach them. Wherever you found this book, you probably read the reviews first.

My point is that if you would kindly leave a review (it only takes 60 seconds. And it's free), you can change other people's lives for the better. Because they will also then read this book.

Thanks.

5. Eat at the same time everyday.

"Timeliness is best in all matters." - Hesiod

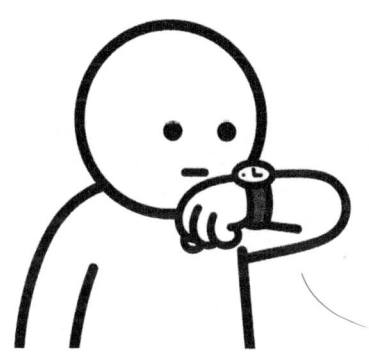

Nature runs on rhythm — sunrise, tides, seasons, flowers. Everything repeats. Your body is part of nature. It too has a cycle, or a rhythm. When you disturb that rhythm, you suffer.

Ever noticed how you get hungry around the same time every day? That's not coincidence. That's your body clock keeping score.

Some people say it's best to wake up naturally, which feels quite… natural. But it's not recommended. In the Vedic culture, the rooster would crow at the optimal time.

Natures' arrangement.

But most of us don't live in a small village with a rooster, so we need a good ol' alarm clock to stay on schedule.

Waking up and going to sleep at consistent times pays off. Your body will adapt to the schedule, and digestion will fire up regularly. Just keep in mind, the schedule doesn't override your hunger. Even if it's 'time to eat.' If you're not hungry, skip it. If you are irregular, the fire will not know when to be ready to digest.

Everyone knows that switching up schedules has a drastic effect. That's why jet lag is a thing; you change the times you usually eat and sleep. Then you feel tired and weird for at least a few days.

Keeping in rhythm also gives you energy and helps you plan your life out. This isn't a self-help book. But if you know your schedule well, it helps to plan and make commitments based on that. You feel more energetic because your body isn't always changing to new bedtimes and dinnertimes.

It can automate itself.

It's muscle memory for your organs. If you do the same thing every day, you get used to it. You do it even without thinking.

Digestion works in exactly the same way. If you respect that clock, digestion becomes automatic. Ignore it, and the whole system drifts out of tune.

A celebrated master of Āyurveda was famous for his strict habits: If his meal wasn't ready by one o'clock, he wouldn't eat at all. Even if it was *one minute* overtime.

You might think that's too much.

I'm not sure he cares.

But look at the rest of nature. The sun doesn't miss a beat. He's never late.

So, that's not always possible for us. Life can be complicated. But as far as possible, if we keep in line with nature, Āyurveda says that we will be happier.

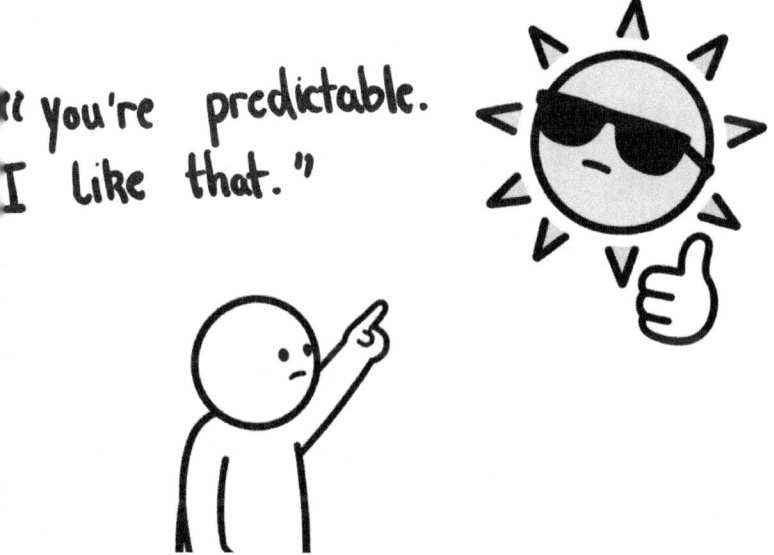

P.S. There was no better place to put this note, but a very imporant part of implementing *all* of the tips in this book is to a) not implement everything all at once, and b) take your time. Doing everything too quickly will shock your body.

6. Burps are your secret weapon.

"There are no quotes about burps by famous people" - Me

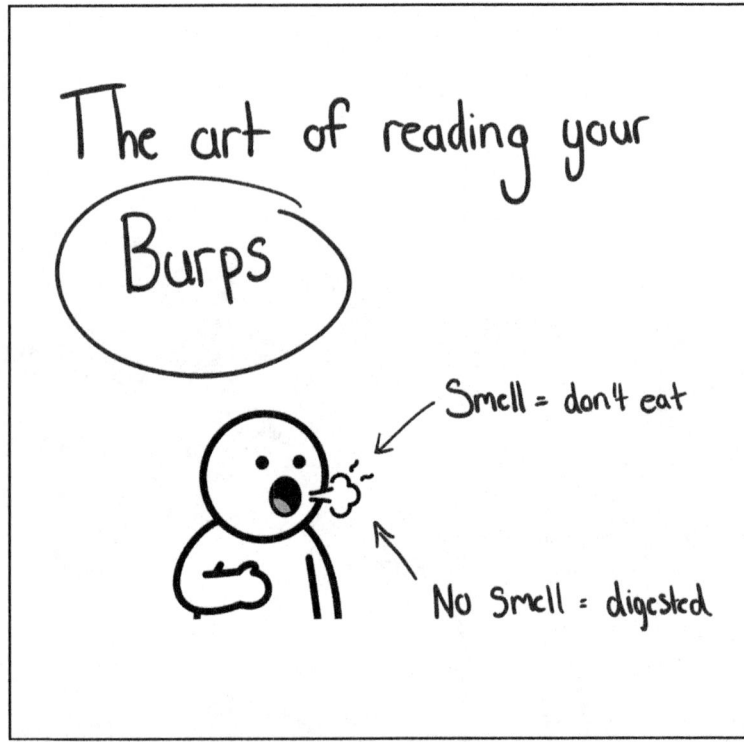

Here's something cool you can try immediately; wait till a few hours after your meal, and you should let out a burp. You'll either taste your last meal when you burp, or it will be flavourless and without smell. If it smells like your last meal, it's still in your stomach. That's why the air from your stomach smells and tastes familiar.. If it's free from any smell or taste, congratulations: your digestive fire should be on very soon.

Before you eat, you should feel the fire of hunger in your

stomach. As you eat, that fiery feeling calms down. There are five stages (I already mentioned them):

Hungry, less hunger, satisfied (no hunger, no fullness), full, and overeaten. We don't want to ever reach the fifth stage.

Well, maybe you do.

But what if I told you stopping just before even the fourth stage was the best? It might be a bit hard to swallow (no pun intended). Because we usually equate fullness with satisfaction. When you feel full, it means your body is telling you to stop eating. You've reached your limit, but being *full* isn't always ideal. The stomach needs ¼ of its space *free* for air flow.

For steady energy and a feeling of lightness and clarity, opt for slightly less than full. The feeling of fullness itself can be a distraction. It's a sensation that brings a certain degree of discomfort and heaviness.

The good thing is that your body will tell you when you should stop eating. It's called burping. Yeah, that thing your mother told you not to do.

Let's go back to our ratio of air-food-water in the stomach. The air part is important here. When you get the right mix of food, water, and air, your gut sends a burp. This means the balance is just right. Don't believe it? Try eating with more focus and at a relaxed pace. You'll find that towards the end of your meal, just as you start to feel full, the burp will come. Like clockwork.

That burp is nature's signal to stop eating. If you eat just one ounce more than that, you'll feel indigestion. It depends on how much you overdo it. The difference between adhering to the burp and not is like the difference between night and day.

Your body communicates to you. When you feel full, your stomach is sending signals through your nervous system that it's at its capacity. When you're hungry, your mind meditates on food, and your tongue salivates when food is in sight. Pain signals that one should avoid something. The burp is another sign. It's not random. It's just one that people generally don't know about.

But now you do, so that's cool.

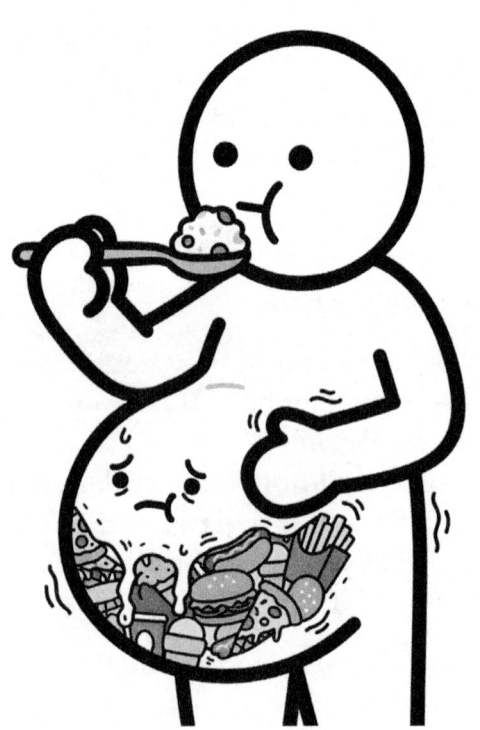

Just hear that guy out...

7. Don't eat at night.

"Last night I dreamt I ate a ten pound marshmallow. When I woke up the pillow was gone." - Tommy Cooper

"Oh no, he's going for the family dinner. Leave that alone!"

Well, sorry, it's gotta go.

Here's a fun fact: your digestion functions like the sun as it rises and sets.

Plants bloom in the daylight, and humans and animals awaken. And so does your stomach.

When the sun is low in the sky, either in the morning

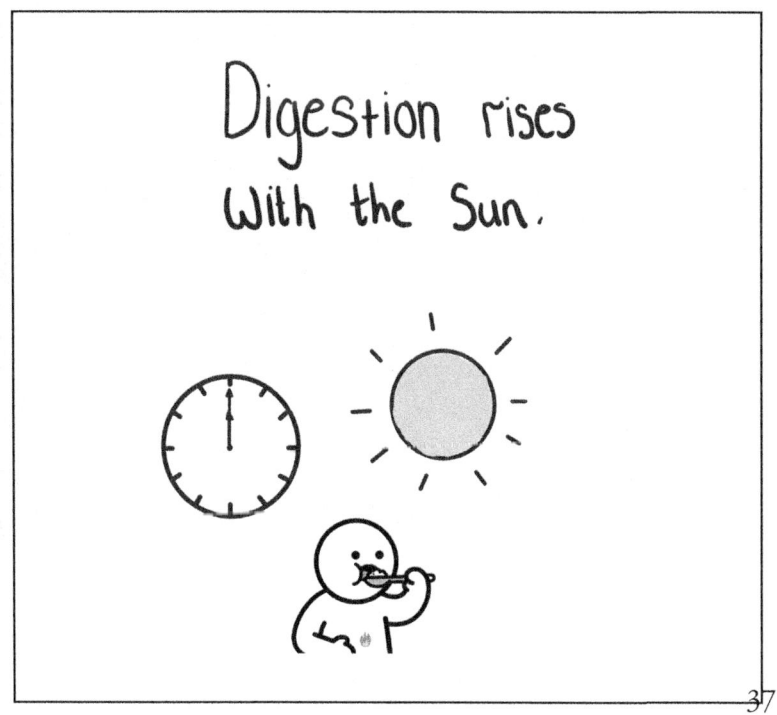

or the evening, your digestion functions poorly. And when the sun is at its highest point, digestion is also at its strongest. That's why, traditionally, lunch is the biggest meal, and breakfast is relatively light. But the unfortunate mistake many people make is that they eat heavy meals, or at all, at night. When the sun sets, your body is already winding down for bed.

In general, people sleep at night. It's natural. It's not the time for working. There's no light. We need light to work. So, it's nature's way of saying "stop, sleep," but we don't listen. We eat. And if we go against nature, we suffer.

You can test this for yourself. You'll find that your hunger is usually weak in the morning and at night. It gets

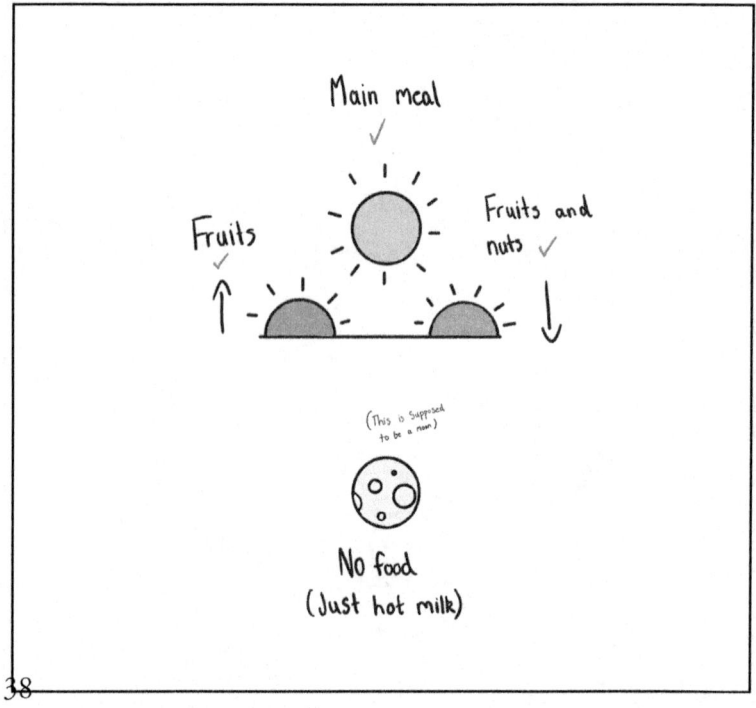

voracious during the daytime.

You wouldn't start cooking dinner when the kitchen fire is dying out — but that's what eating late is.

According to Āyurveda, the only thing that digests well at night is hot milk. In fact, your body releases special enzymes to digest hot milk. If you're feeling hungry, a couple of glasses of hot milk will satisfy you.

Try this if you don't believe me: eat a meal at night. When you wake up, notice how you feel. Then, compare that to a morning after just a glass of hot milk.

The difference speaks for itself.

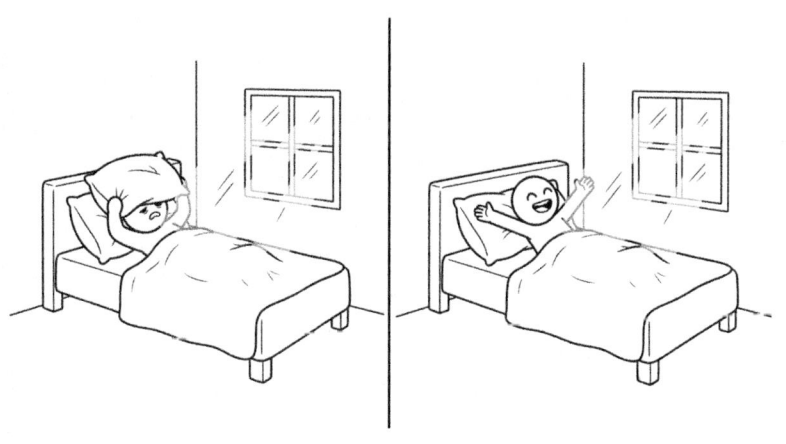

A rough estimate of your before and after

8. Good sleep.

"Happiness and unhappiness, nourishment, good physical strength and debility, sexual prowess and intimacy, and ignorance, life, and death—all are dependent on sleep."

– Ashtanga Hridayam

This might be the shortest point in the book. Like, it will only take a paragraph. But it's one of the most important. Āyurveda points out that good rest is vital. Without it, your organs, especially your digestion, can't work properly. And so, all the other tips in this short book won't be very helpful if you don't get enough rest.

If you feel tired, it's difficult to do things, right? Let's say you like to run. Or cook. Or any physical activity. If you're exhausted, you can't put much energy or time into that activity, even if you love it.

Your stomach feels exactly like you do. That little guy *loves* to digest. Usually. If you treat him right. But he won't be able to do his job if he feels tired.

So good rest is important because if you're tired, so is your stomach. And if he's tired, your digestion is weak.

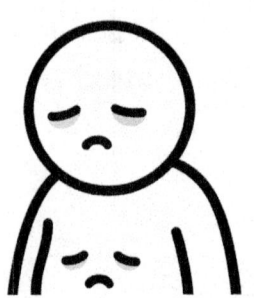

When your digestion is weak, the source of energy, a.k.a. food, will not be well digested, which leads to more tiredness.

Cycle of life, baby.

The amount of sleep you need depends on you. It's not like 8 or 7 hours is the golden standard. Some people do well on 6, some well on 9. If you feel energetic and rested, then however many hours it took to feel good is the right amount of sleep for you. It depends alot on the quantity of food you ate and the extent of your physical or mental effort.

A wise old saying is "early to bed, early to rise, makes a man healthy, wealthy, and wise."

It took a bit longer than a paragraph. I'm not sorry about it.

This stuff is important.

9. Food as a medicine

"When diet is wrong, medicine is of no use. When diet is correct, medicine is of no need."

- Ancient Āyurvedic proverb

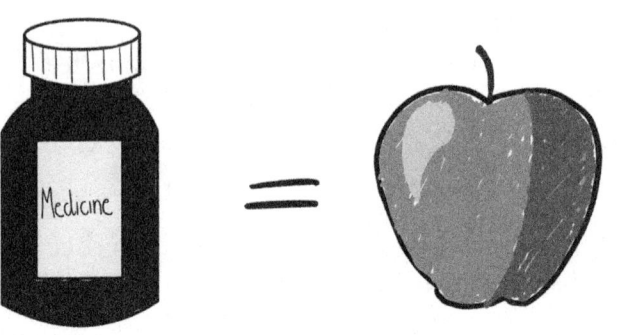

Most people see food as pleasure. Or escape. Or survival. But food is medicine. I won't cover how different food affects the body and mind here. The habits we discussed in this short book are the fastest and most lasting ways to achieve good health, as per Āyurveda.

Food, and the way of consuming it, is medicine. If we consume food for enjoyment, we tend to overeat. Or eat when it's not the right time. That causes problems.

When we see food as medicine, we do what's required (like the methods I mentioned in this book) to keep ourselves fit.

Food is also a 'double-edged sword' because it is both the cause of health *and* disease. If we eat well, we become strong and healthy. If we eat incorrectly, we receive the opposite result.

Some people see food as an escape from suffering. The delicious tastes and familiar smells that remind us of 'mammas' cooking' bring us joy.

The irony is that eating food in a wrong way causes more suffering by creating disease.

When we learn *how* to eat, our very existence can become blissful, clear, and inspired. If we don't learn how to eat, our system gets glued up by undigested waste. A clogged mind can't think. A tired body can't move. We miss life when health fails — the events, the joy, the focus. Eating correctly isn't just following rules and hoping for a better future. It's a remedy for most of our non-hereditary bodily pains that works quickly.

When someone offers you seconds, see it as an attack on your wellbeing. Don't go crazy, but understand the consequences of going against nature.

There are *many* downsides when choosing to ignore Āyurveda. On the flipside, many get good results from following it.

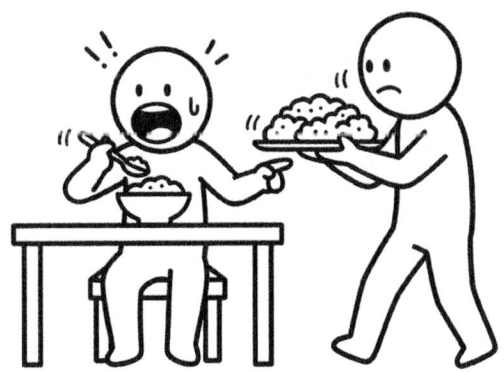

10. Battle with your mind.

"For one who has conquered his mind, a mind is the best of friends, but for one who has failed to do so, his very mind will be the greatest enemy."

-Krishna, Bhagavad-gita

Your biggest enemy on the path to better health is your own mind. This isn't a book about meditation. But it is closely tied to knowing our minds and working to break bad habits.

The world around us conditions us to consume without consideration. Advertisements attack us, making food look too tasty. We cannot say no.

In the UK, there's even a fast-food delivery company called "Just eat." That mantra, much like clever propaganda, urges us to overlook our bodies. As in, "Just eat, you animal." But is eating the only consideration? What about if we are even hungry at all?

Few people know the secrets of Āyurveda. Much of modern nutrition advice misses the point. They talk how many times a day we should eat, and what we should eat. But they rarely consider if we are even hungry at all. In fact, Āyurveda tells us what we already know; hunger is the sign that we should eat.

But we have become so misled that when we feel hunger, we think it's a sign we're about die. In fact, we pay so little attention to our digestive health that few people ever experience hunger at all. We think of hunger as something negative, something that should be avoided at all costs. Like hunger is only for 'poor people' who can't afford to eat so much.

Yet hunger is our friend. It's our signal that we are ready to eat. If we eat at that time, we'll be healthy, strong, and happy. We even relish the taste of the food more.

You don't need a certificate to know you're hungry. You know. But our lives get so busy, and food is so good and convenient that we eat things just to taste them.

> Your mind is against you. He'll try to talk you into things you will regret.
>
> That rascal doesn't eat. Don't listen to him.

We don't consider how our bodies will handle what we consume, nor do we know what will happen as a result.

The Āyurveda says that almost all disease is a result of poor digestion.

Think about it.

Disease is inevitable, yes, because that's nature. Our bodies are fragile. But why should we risk more than necessary?

The mind will try to fight you. It will say, "c'mon, take another one. One more bite. It was so good. You'll try this 'Āyurveda' stuff tomorrow, or next week. Worry about it later. You're with friends! Family! You can't be rude. Eat it up. You're bored, you're sad, eat."

But you can say no. Every time you do, you get stronger. The more you say no and adapt your life to the principles in this book, the stronger your mind and body will be.

Āyurveda is a holistic science. By following the rules of Āyurveda, your mind becomes controlled. Character develops. Suffering due to disease and discomfort decreases. Life levels up.

This knowledge will change your life from a health point of view, which helps all the other aspects of your life. You'll likely concentrate better and feel less tired. Many people even notice they need less sleep when digestion improves. They'll save money on wasted meals. They'll gain time to work on the things they love.

Start with your digestion.

Fix that fire, and everything else starts to work again.

To lightness, clarity, and strong digestion,

- Max.

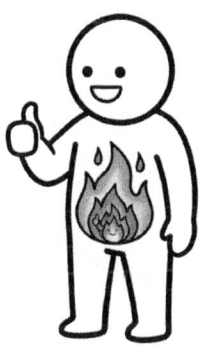

If you're looking to deepen your Ayurveda journey or meet others on the same path, check out our community on skool.com; *The Ayurveda Tree*

If you don't like typing in links, here is a QR code for access:

About the author

Maxim Bishop was a monk for 7 years. He practices the ancient tradition of Vaishnavism.

During his time as a monk he studied the Vedic scriptures, of which Āyurveda is a branch.

He wants to spread the healing knowledge of Āyurveda in ways that are as easy to understand as possible. This book is the first attempt in that endeavor.

He is now married and lives with his wife in London, UK, where he runs his company, Gopi Ayurveda.

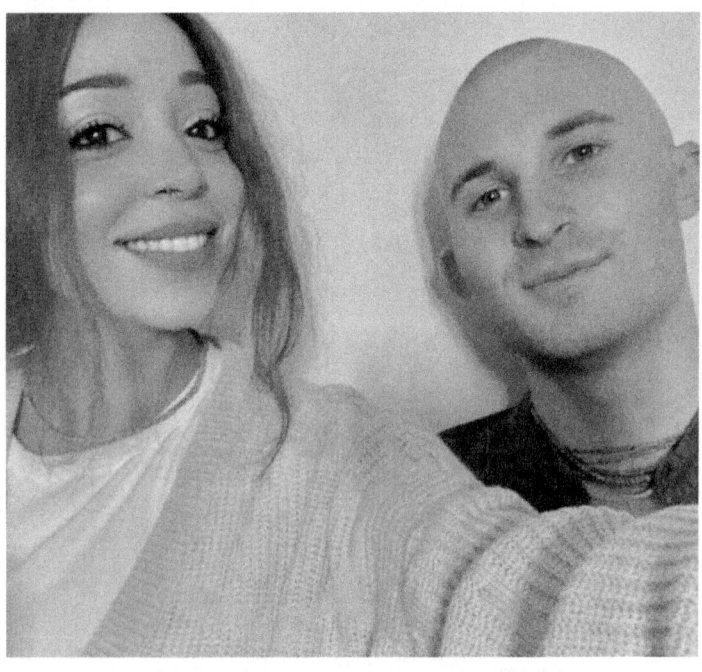

Printed in Dunstable, United Kingdom